FLEXIBILITY AND BALANCE FOR OVER AGES

Finding Harmony: Navigating Life's Twists and Turns with Ease

Scott Meek

Table of Contents

INTRODUCTION

Welcome, dear reader, to the journey ahead. As you crack open this book titled "Flexibility and Balance for All Ages," I want you to know that you're not just flipping through pages; you're embarking on a quest for better movement, enhanced well-being, and perhaps a few laughs along the way.

Now, before we delve into the nitty-gritty of muscles, joints, and balancing acts, let's take a moment to sit back, relax, and ponder the wonder that is the human body. Seriously, have you ever stopped to marvel at the marvel that is you? You, my friend, are a walking, talking masterpiece of biology, chemistry, and a touch of cosmic stardust. Your body can bend, twist, stretch, and balance in ways that would make a Cirque du Soleil performer envious (okay, maybe not all of us, but you get the gist).

But here's the thing – as magnificent as our bodies are, they sometimes need a little TLC. And that's where flexibility and balance come into play. Whether you're a sprightly youngster or a seasoned senior, maintaining flexibility and balance is crucial for navigating this crazy thing we call life. Trust me, I get it. Life can throw some unexpected curveballs – from dodging runaway shopping carts at the grocery store to attempting to gracefully dismount from a wobbly office chair (spoiler alert: it never ends well).

So, why should you care about flexibility and balance? Well, my friend, let me tell you a little secret – they're the unsung heroes of everyday movement. Think about it: every time you reach for that jar of pickles on the top shelf or attempt to tie your shoelaces without face-planting, you're relying on your body's flexibility and balance to get the job done. And let's not forget about those moments when life throws us a curveball (or a banana peel, whichever comes first). Whether it's dodging a rogue soccer ball or navigating a crowded subway car during rush hour, having a solid foundation of flexibility and balance can mean the difference between a graceful save and a not-so-graceful tumble.

But here's the kicker – flexibility and balance aren't just about avoiding embarrassing spills (although that's certainly a bonus). They're also about living life to the fullest, no matter your age or stage. Whether you're a wide-eyed child discovering the joys of cartwheels and handstands, a busy adult juggling work, family, and everything in between, or a wise elder gracefully navigating the golden years, flexibility and balance are your trusty companions on the journey of life.

Now, I know what you're thinking – "But wait, isn't flexibility just for contortionists and gymnasts? And isn't balance something only tightrope walkers and circus performers need?" Not so, my friend. Flexibility and balance are for everyone – yes, even you. Whether you're a seasoned athlete or a self-proclaimed couch potato, there's always room to improve your flexibility and balance. And trust me, your body will thank you for it.

In this book, we'll dive headfirst into the fascinating world of flexibility and balance, exploring everything from the science behind stretching to the art of staying upright on two feet (or one foot, if you're feeling adventurous). But more than that, we'll embark on a journey of self-discovery, empowerment, and maybe even a few moments of self-deprecating humor (because let's face it, we've all had our fair share of clumsy mishaps).

So, my fellow adventurer, I invite you to join me on this quest for greater flexibility, better balance, and a whole lot of laughs along the way. Whether you're flipping through these pages out of curiosity, desperation, or sheer boredom (hey, no judgment here), know that you're not alone. We're in this together, navigating the twists and turns of life one stretch, one wobble, and one belly laugh at a time.

So buckle up, my friend. The journey ahead promises to be a wild ride. But I have a feeling it'll be one heck of an adventure.

Let's do this.

Warmest regards,

UNDERSTANDING THE IMPORTANCE OF FLEXIBILITY AND BALANCE

Flexibility and balance are not just buzzwords in the realm of fitness; they are pillars of overall well-being that support every stage of life. From the playground to the boardroom and beyond, the benefits of maintaining optimal flexibility and balance extend far beyond the confines of the gym. In this chapter, we will explore the profound importance of flexibility and balance across age groups, shedding light on their myriad benefits and why they should be prioritized in your daily routine.

Benefits for Every Age Group

Flexibility and balance are two sides of the same coin, each contributing to the overall harmony and functionality of the human body. Let's take a closer look at how these fundamental components of fitness benefit individuals of all ages.

- **Children and Adolescents**

As budding explorers of the world around them, children and adolescents rely heavily on flexibility and balance to navigate the physical challenges they encounter daily. From climbing trees to mastering the monkey bars, these young adventurers rely on their bodies' flexibility to stretch, reach, and explore with ease.

Furthermore, flexibility and balance play a crucial role in the development of motor skills during childhood and adolescence. As children engage in various physical activities, they are constantly refining their coordination, proprioception, and spatial awareness – all of which are essential components of balance.

By incorporating activities that promote flexibility and balance into their daily routine, children and adolescents can lay the foundation for a lifetime of good health and physical literacy. Whether it's participating in sports, dance classes, or simply engaging in active play, fostering flexibility and balance during these formative years sets the stage for a lifetime of physical well-being.

- **Adults**

In the hustle and bustle of adult life, it's easy to overlook the importance of flexibility and balance amidst the demands of work, family, and other responsibilities. However, neglecting these fundamental aspects of fitness can have far-reaching consequences for overall health and quality of life.

For adults, maintaining flexibility and balance is essential for preventing injuries, improving posture, and enhancing performance in everyday activities. Whether it's bending down to tie your shoes, lifting groceries, or sitting at a desk for extended periods, flexibility and balance are key to moving with ease and grace throughout the day.

Furthermore, as we age, flexibility and balance become even more critical for maintaining independence and reducing the risk of falls and injuries. By incorporating regular stretching exercises and balance training into their routine, adults can mitigate the effects of aging on their musculoskeletal system and preserve their mobility and vitality well into their later years.

- **Older Adults**

For older adults, flexibility and balance take on even greater significance as they navigate the challenges of aging and age-related changes in physical function. As muscle mass decreases, joints become stiffer, and balance deteriorates, older adults are at an increased risk of falls and fractures – a leading cause of morbidity and mortality in this population. However, by prioritizing activities that promote flexibility and balance, older adults can significantly reduce their risk of falls and maintain their independence and quality of life. Exercises such as yoga, tai chi, and Pilates are particularly beneficial for improving flexibility, balance, and proprioception in older adults, helping them stay active, mobile, and engaged in life.

Moreover, flexibility and balance training can have a profound impact on cognitive function and emotional well-being in older adults. Research has shown that regular exercise, including activities that target flexibility and balance, can improve cognitive function, reduce the risk of dementia, and alleviate symptoms of depression and anxiety.

THE SCIENCE BEHIND FLEXIBILITY

Flexibility is not just about touching your toes or doing the splits; it's a complex interplay of anatomical structures, physiological processes, and environmental factors that determine the range of motion in our joints. In this chapter, we will delve into the science behind flexibility, exploring the intricate workings of our muscles, joints, and connective tissues, as well as how flexibility changes with age and the various factors that influence it.

Anatomy of Flexibility: Muscles, Joints, and Connective Tissues

To understand flexibility, we must first unravel the intricate anatomy of the musculoskeletal system – the framework that supports our bodies and enables movement. At the heart of flexibility lies the musculature, a network of muscles and tendons that work in concert to produce movement and maintain posture.

Muscles are the primary drivers of movement, contracting and relaxing to produce the various motions of our bodies. When it comes to flexibility, certain muscles play a particularly crucial role. These include the muscles that span multiple joints, known as articular muscles, as well as the muscles that cross over joints and are responsible for specific movements, known as agonists and antagonists.

In addition to muscles, joints also play a pivotal role in determining flexibility. Joints are the points of articulation between bones, where movement occurs. The structure of a joint – including its shape, size, and the arrangement of ligaments and cartilage – influences its range of motion. For example, ball-and-socket joints, such as the hip joint, have a greater range of motion compared to hinge joints, such as the elbow joint.

Connective tissues, including tendons and ligaments, also contribute to flexibility by providing stability and support to the joints. Tendons connect muscles to bones, transmitting the force generated by muscle contraction to produce movement. Ligaments, on the other hand, connect bones to other bones, reinforcing the joint and preventing excessive movement.

Together, muscles, joints, and connective tissues form a complex network that governs our ability to move and bend. When we engage in activities that promote flexibility, such as stretching exercises, we are not only elongating the muscles but also improving the elasticity of connective tissues and increasing the range of motion in our joints.

How Flexibility Changes with Age

As we journey through life, our bodies undergo a myriad of changes that impact our flexibility. From the exuberance of youth to the wisdom of old age, each stage of life brings its own unique challenges and opportunities for growth – both physical and emotional.

During childhood and adolescence, the body is in a state of rapid growth and development, with flexibility reaching its peak during this period. Children are naturally more flexible than adults due to factors such as lower muscle mass, greater elasticity of connective tissues, and less resistance from bones and joints.

However, as we transition into adulthood, flexibility begins to decline gradually. This decline is influenced by various factors, including changes in muscle elasticity, loss of water content in connective tissues, and alterations in joint structure and function. Additionally, lifestyle factors such as sedentary behavior, poor posture, and lack of physical activity can exacerbate the loss of flexibility over time.

By the time we reach older adulthood, flexibility may become significantly impaired, leading to stiffness, joint pain, and reduced range of motion. This decline in flexibility is not inevitable, however. With regular exercise and targeted stretching routines, older adults can maintain and even improve their flexibility, thereby enhancing their mobility and quality of life.

Factors Affecting Flexibility

Flexibility is influenced by a multitude of factors, ranging from genetics and anatomy to lifestyle and environmental factors. While some of these factors are beyond our control, others can be modified through conscious effort and behavior change.

Genetics play a significant role in determining an individual's baseline level of flexibility. Some people are naturally more flexible than others due to genetic variations in muscle and connective tissue composition, joint structure, and other biological factors. However, while genetics may predispose us to a certain degree of flexibility, it does not necessarily dictate our ultimate potential. With consistent effort and dedication, anyone can improve their flexibility regardless of their genetic predisposition.

Anatomy also plays a crucial role in determining flexibility. Factors such as joint structure, muscle length, and the arrangement of connective tissues can influence an individual's range of motion. For example, individuals with longer limbs and more mobile joints may have a greater range of motion compared to those with shorter limbs and less flexible joints.

Lifestyle and environmental factors also have a significant impact on flexibility. Sedentary behavior, prolonged sitting, and lack of physical activity can lead to muscle tightness and stiffness, reducing flexibility over time. Conversely, regular exercise, stretching, and mobility work can improve flexibility and prevent age-related declines in range of motion.

flexibility is a multifaceted concept that encompasses the interplay of anatomical structures, physiological processes, and environmental factors. By understanding the science behind flexibility and the factors that influence it, we can empower ourselves to take proactive steps to improve our flexibility and enhance our overall health and well-being. Through targeted stretching routines, regular exercise, and mindful movement practices, we can unlock our body's full potential and embrace a life of greater mobility, vitality, and resilience.

ASSESSING YOUR CURRENT FLEXIBILITY AND BALANCE

Understanding your current level of flexibility and balance is essential for designing an effective training program tailored to your needs and goals. By conducting a thorough self-assessment, you can identify areas of strength and weakness, establish baseline measurements, and track your progress over time. In this chapter, we'll explore self-assessment techniques and setting baseline measurements to help you evaluate your current flexibility and balance effectively.

Self-Assessment Techniques

Self-assessment techniques are valuable tools for gaining insight into your flexibility and balance capabilities. These techniques involve observing and analyzing your body's movements, range of motion, and stability to identify areas for improvement. Here are some effective self-assessment techniques to consider:

- **Joint Mobility Assessment**: Start by assessing the mobility of key joints in your body, such as the shoulders, hips, knees, and ankles. Perform simple range of motion exercises for each joint, such as shoulder circles, hip rotations, knee bends, and ankle circles. Pay attention to any restrictions or limitations in movement and note areas that feel tight or restricted.

- **Static Stretching Test**: Conduct a series of static stretching exercises to assess your flexibility in major muscle groups. Focus on areas commonly associated with tightness, such as the hamstrings, quadriceps, calves, chest, and shoulders. Hold each stretch for 20-30 seconds and assess the range of motion and sensation of tension or discomfort. Note any differences in flexibility between the left and right sides of your body.

- **Balance Exercises**: Perform a variety of balance exercises to evaluate your stability and proprioception. Start with simple exercises such as standing on one leg or balancing on a stability ball, then progress to more challenging movements as you feel comfortable. Pay attention to your ability to maintain balance and stability, and note any difficulty or instability you experience.

- **Functional Movement Screening**: Consider conducting a functional movement screening to assess your overall movement patterns and identify any asymmetries or dysfunctions. This screening typically involves a series of movements such as squats, lunges, and overhead reaches, which are evaluated for proper alignment, stability, and coordination. Look for any compensations or imbalances that may indicate areas for improvement.

- **Postural Analysis**: Take a closer look at your posture to identify any postural deviations or imbalances that may affect your flexibility and balance. Stand in front of a mirror and observe your alignment from the front, side, and back. Look for signs of forward head posture, rounded shoulders, excessive curvature of the spine, or pelvic tilt. These observations can provide valuable insights into areas of weakness or tightness that may contribute to poor flexibility and balance.

By incorporating these self-assessment techniques into your routine, you can gain a better understanding of your current flexibility and balance levels and identify areas for improvement. Remember to approach self-assessment with an open mind and without judgment, using the information gathered to inform your training program and set realistic goals for progress.

Setting Baseline Measurements

Once you've completed your self-assessment, it's important to establish baseline measurements to track your progress over time. Baseline measurements provide a starting point for your flexibility and balance journey and serve as a reference point for monitoring improvements and identifying areas of focus. Here are some key baseline measurements to consider:

- **Flexibility Measurements**: Measure your flexibility using specific tests or assessments for major muscle groups and joints. For example, you can use a sit-and-reach test to measure hamstring flexibility, a shoulder flexion test to assess shoulder mobility, or a calf flexibility test to evaluate ankle flexibility. Record your measurements in inches or centimeters to track changes over time.

- **Balance Assessments**: Conduct balance assessments to evaluate your stability and proprioception. This may include tests such as the single-leg stance test, tandem stance test, or dynamic balance exercises such as walking heel-to-toe or standing on a foam pad with eyes closed. Measure the duration you can maintain each position or the number of successful repetitions to establish baseline scores.

- **Functional Movement Screening Scores**: If you've performed a functional movement screening, record your scores for each movement pattern or exercise. This may involve assigning a numerical score based on the quality of movement or noting any compensations or dysfunctions observed during the screening process. Use these scores to track changes in movement quality and identify areas for improvement.

- **Postural Analysis Findings**: Document your postural analysis findings, including observations of any postural deviations or imbalances. Take photographs or video recordings from multiple angles to capture your posture from different perspectives. Use these images as a visual reference to track changes in alignment and posture over time.

- **Subjective Feedback**: Lastly, don't forget to include subjective feedback from your self-assessment in your baseline measurements. Take note of any sensations of tightness, discomfort, or instability you experience during exercises or movements. Use this feedback to inform your training program and set goals for improvement in specific areas.

Once you've established baseline measurements for your flexibility and balance, be sure to revisit them regularly to track your progress and adjust your training program accordingly. Celebrate your achievements along the way, and remember that progress may not always be linear. With dedication, consistency, and a commitment to self-improvement, you can enhance your flexibility and balance and unlock your full potential for health and well-being. assessing your current flexibility and balance is the first step towards creating a tailored training program that addresses your individual needs and goals. By incorporating self-assessment techniques and setting baseline measurements, you can gain valuable insights into your strengths and weaknesses and track your progress over time. Armed with this information, you can design a targeted training program that optimizes your flexibility, enhances your balance, and improves your overall quality of life. So, take the time to assess where you are today, set realistic goals for tomorrow, and embark on your journey towards greater flexibility and balance with confidence and determination.

FLEXIBILITY TRAINING TECHNIQUES

Flexibility is a fundamental component of overall fitness and plays a crucial role in enhancing athletic performance, reducing the risk of injury, and improving daily function. Flexibility training techniques encompass a variety of methods and approaches aimed at increasing range of motion, reducing muscle tension, and improving joint mobility. In this chapter, we'll explore three key flexibility training techniques: stretching exercises, yoga and Pilates, and flexibility training programs.

Stretching Exercises

Stretching exercises are perhaps the most well-known and commonly used method for improving flexibility. Stretching involves lengthening muscles and soft tissues to increase their elasticity and range of motion. There are several different types of stretching exercises, each with its own benefits and applications.

- **Static Stretching**: Static stretching involves holding a stretch in a comfortable position for a set period, typically 20-30 seconds. This type of stretching helps improve flexibility by gradually elongating muscles and increasing joint mobility. Common static stretches include hamstring stretches, calf stretches, quadriceps stretches, and shoulder stretches.

- **Dynamic Stretching**: Dynamic stretching involves moving joints and muscles through a full range of motion in a controlled manner. Unlike static stretching, dynamic stretching is performed in a rhythmic and repetitive fashion, often mimicking movements used in sports or activities. Dynamic stretches help improve flexibility, mobility, and muscle activation while also serving as a warm-up for physical activity.

- **Proprioceptive Neuromuscular Facilitation (PNF)**: PNF stretching techniques involve a combination of passive stretching and muscle contraction to enhance flexibility. This technique typically involves stretching a muscle to its end range, contracting the muscle against resistance for several seconds, and then relaxing and stretching the muscle further. PNF stretching is believed to improve flexibility more rapidly than other stretching methods and is commonly used in rehabilitation and sports performance settings.

- **Active Isolated Stretching (AIS)**: AIS is a dynamic stretching technique that focuses on isolated muscle groups. It involves actively contracting one muscle while stretching its antagonist muscle to promote reciprocal inhibition and increase flexibility. AIS is often used by athletes and fitness enthusiasts to improve flexibility, mobility, and athletic performance.

When incorporating stretching exercises into your flexibility training routine, it's essential to warm up the body beforehand to prepare muscles and joints for stretching. Start with gentle movements and dynamic stretches to increase blood flow and flexibility, then progress to static or PNF stretches to target specific muscle groups. Remember to breathe deeply and relax into each stretch, avoiding bouncing or jerking movements that can lead to injury.

Yoga and Pilates for Flexibility

Yoga and Pilates are two mind-body practices that emphasize flexibility, strength, and balance through a series of controlled movements and poses. Both disciplines offer a holistic approach to improving flexibility, incorporating elements of stretching, strengthening, and mindfulness to promote overall well-being.

- **Yoga**: Yoga is an ancient practice originating from India that focuses on physical postures (asanas), breath control (pranayama), and meditation (dhyana) to promote health and relaxation. Many yoga poses are designed to improve flexibility by stretching muscles, opening joints, and increasing range of motion. Common yoga poses for flexibility include downward-facing dog, forward fold, seated forward bend, and pigeon pose. Yoga classes often incorporate a variety of poses, sequences, and breathing techniques to enhance flexibility, reduce stress, and cultivate mindfulness.

- **Pilates**: Pilates is a system of exercises developed by Joseph Pilates in the early 20th century to improve physical fitness, rehabilitation, and performance. Pilates focuses on core strength, stability, and body awareness through a series of controlled movements performed on a mat or specialized equipment such as a reformer or Cadillac. Pilates exercises often involve dynamic movements that simultaneously stretch and strengthen muscles, promoting flexibility, mobility, and postural alignment. Common Pilates exercises for flexibility include the hundred, spine stretch forward, saw, and swan dive.

Both yoga and Pilates offer a safe and effective way to improve flexibility, balance, and overall fitness for individuals of all ages and fitness levels. Whether you prefer the flowing sequences of yoga or the precise movements of Pilates, incorporating these practices into your flexibility training routine can help you achieve your flexibility goals while also enhancing strength, stability, and mental clarity.

Flexibility Training Programs

Flexibility training programs are structured plans designed to systematically improve flexibility and range of motion over time. These programs often incorporate a combination of stretching exercises, yoga or Pilates classes, and targeted mobility drills to address specific areas of tightness or restriction. Here are some key components of effective flexibility training programs:

- **Individualized Approach**: A successful flexibility training program takes into account individual differences in flexibility, mobility, and biomechanics. Tailor your program to address your unique needs and goals, focusing on areas of tightness or restriction that may be limiting your flexibility and performance.

- **Progressive Overload**: Like any fitness program, flexibility training should incorporate progressive overload to promote adaptation and improvement. Gradually increase the intensity, duration, and frequency of stretching exercises over time to challenge your muscles and stimulate gains in flexibility.

- **Variety and Specificity**: Incorporate a variety of stretching exercises, yoga poses, and Pilates movements into your flexibility training program to target different muscle groups and movement patterns. Focus on specific areas of tightness or restriction while also addressing overall flexibility and mobility.

- **Consistency and Frequency**: Consistency is key when it comes to flexibility training. Aim to stretch regularly, ideally on a daily basis, to maintain and improve flexibility over time. Incorporate stretching exercises into your warm-up and cool-down routines, as well as standalone stretching sessions focused on specific areas of concern.

- **Recovery and Rest**: Allow time for rest and recovery between flexibility training sessions to prevent overuse injuries and promote muscle recovery. Listen to your body's signals and avoid pushing through pain or discomfort during stretching exercises. Incorporate restorative practices such as foam rolling, massage, or gentle yoga to aid in recovery and reduce muscle soreness.

By following these principles and guidelines, you can create a comprehensive flexibility training program that addresses your individual needs and goals. Remember to listen to your body, progress at your own pace, and stay consistent with your training to achieve lasting improvements in flexibility, mobility, and overall well-being. flexibility training techniques such as stretching exercises, yoga, and Pilates offer effective ways to improve flexibility, mobility, and range of motion. By incorporating these techniques into your flexibility training routine and following a structured flexibility training program, you can enhance your physical performance, reduce the risk of injury, and improve your overall quality of life. So, whether you're a seasoned athlete looking to optimize performance or someone simply seeking to move more freely and comfortably, flexibility training has something to offer for everyone. Embrace the journey towards greater flexibility, and enjoy the benefits of a body that moves with ease and grace.

IMPROVING BALANCE

Balance is a fundamental aspect of physical function that influences our ability to perform daily activities, participate in sports and recreational activities, and reduce the risk of falls and injuries. As we age, maintaining and improving balance becomes increasingly important for preserving mobility and independence. In this chapter, we'll explore three key approaches to improving balance: balance exercises for adults, Tai Chi and Qigong, and balance training programs.

Balance Exercises for Adults

Balance exercises for adults are designed to challenge stability, proprioception, and coordination to improve balance and reduce the risk of falls. These exercises often target the core muscles, lower body strength, and neuromuscular control to enhance stability and postural control. Here are some effective balance exercises for adults to incorporate into their fitness routine:

- **Single-Leg Stance**: Stand on one leg with the opposite foot lifted slightly off the ground. Focus on maintaining your balance while keeping your hips level and core engaged. Hold this position for 30 seconds to one minute, then switch legs. To increase the challenge, try closing your eyes or performing small movements with your arms or head while balancing.

- **Tandem Stance**: Stand with one foot directly in front of the other, heel to toe, as if walking on a tightrope. Keep your arms relaxed at your sides and your gaze focused on a fixed point in front of you. Hold this position for 30 seconds to one minute, then switch sides. Focus on maintaining your balance and stability throughout the exercise.

- **Balance Board Drills**: Use a balance board or wobble board to challenge your balance and proprioception. Stand on the board with your feet hip-width apart and engage your core muscles to stabilize your body. Rock the board from side to side or front to back while maintaining your balance. As you become more comfortable, try performing exercises such as squats, lunges, or single-leg stands on the balance board to further challenge your stability.

- **Standing Heel Raises**: Stand with your feet hip-width apart and lift your heels off the ground, rising up onto the balls of your feet. Hold this position for a few seconds, then lower your heels back down to the ground. Repeat for 10-15 repetitions, focusing on maintaining your balance and control throughout the movement.

- **Clock Reach**: Stand on one leg with your arms extended out to your sides. Imagine yourself standing in the center of a clock, with 12 o'clock directly in front of you. Slowly reach your arms forward and overhead to touch 12 o'clock, then return to the starting position. Repeat the movement, reaching towards different points on the clock (e.g., 3 o'clock, 6 o'clock, 9 o'clock) to challenge your balance and stability from different angles.

Incorporate these balance exercises into your regular fitness routine, aiming to perform them at least two to three times per week. Start with easier variations of each exercise and gradually increase the difficulty as you become more proficient. Consistency is key when it comes to improving balance, so make it a habit to include balance exercises in your workouts to maintain and enhance stability and mobility.

Tai Chi and Qigong for Balance

Tai Chi and Qigong are ancient mind-body practices originating from China that emphasize slow, flowing movements, deep breathing, and mindfulness to promote health and well-being. These practices have been shown to improve balance, strength, flexibility, and mental clarity, making them ideal for individuals looking to enhance their balance and overall quality of life.

- **Tai Chi**: Tai Chi, also known as Tai Chi Chuan, is a martial art characterized by slow, deliberate movements performed in a continuous, flowing manner. Tai Chi sequences, or forms, typically consist of a series of movements that flow seamlessly from one to the next, incorporating shifting weight, controlled breathing, and mindful awareness of body alignment and posture. Tai Chi has been extensively studied for its health benefits, including improvements in balance, mobility, and fall prevention.

- **Qigong**: Qigong, pronounced "Chee-gong," is a holistic practice that combines movement, meditation, and breath work to cultivate qi, or vital energy, within the body. Qigong exercises often involve gentle, repetitive movements performed in coordination with deep breathing and focused attention. Qigong practices vary widely, ranging from simple standing exercises to more complex sequences that integrate movement with visualization and intention. Like Tai Chi, Qigong has been shown to improve balance, reduce stress, and enhance overall well-being.

Both Tai Chi and Qigong offer accessible and low-impact ways to improve balance and mobility for people of all ages and fitness levels. Whether practiced as a standalone activity or incorporated into a broader fitness routine, these mind-body practices can provide valuable benefits for enhancing balance, reducing fall risk, and promoting overall health and vitality.

Balance Training Programs

Balance training programs are structured plans designed to systematically improve balance and stability through a combination of exercises and activities. These programs often incorporate a variety of balance exercises, Tai Chi or Qigong practices, and functional movements to address specific balance deficits and enhance overall stability. Here are some key components of effective balance training programs:

- **Progressive Challenge**: A successful balance training program should gradually increase the difficulty and complexity of exercises over time to challenge balance and stability. Start with basic balance exercises and progress to more advanced variations as you become more proficient.

- **Variety and Adaptability**: Incorporate a variety of balance exercises and activities into your training program to target different aspects of balance and stability. Include exercises that challenge static balance, dynamic balance, and reactive balance to improve overall stability and reduce fall risk.

- **Functional Movements**: Incorporate functional movements and activities into your balance training program to improve balance in real-world scenarios. Focus on exercises that mimic everyday activities such as walking, climbing stairs, and reaching for objects to enhance functional balance and mobility.

- **Individualized Approach**: Tailor your balance training program to address your specific needs and goals, taking into account factors such as age, fitness level, and any existing balance deficits or injuries. Modify exercises as needed to accommodate individual abilities and limitations, and progress at a pace that feels comfortable and safe.

- **Consistency and Persistence**: Like any fitness program, consistency and persistence are essential for achieving results with balance training. Aim to incorporate balance exercises into your routine at least two to three times per week, and make it a habit to practice Tai Chi or Qigong regularly to maintain and enhance balance and stability over time.

By following these principles and guidelines, you can create a comprehensive balance training program that improves stability, reduces fall risk, and enhances overall quality of life. Remember to listen to your body, progress at your own pace, and stay consistent with your training to achieve lasting improvements in balance and mobility. Improving balance is essential for maintaining mobility, independence, and overall quality of life, especially as we age. By incorporating balance exercises, Tai Chi and Qigong practices, and structured balance training programs into your fitness routine, you can enhance stability, reduce fall risk, and promote optimal physical function and well-being. So, whether you're a fitness enthusiast looking to enhance athletic performance or someone simply seeking to move with greater confidence and ease, balance training offers valuable benefits for people of all ages and abilities. Embrace the journey towards better balance, and enjoy the rewards of a body that moves with grace, stability, and vitality.

ENHANCING FLEXIBILITY THROUGH STRETCHING

Flexibility is not a static attribute; it's a quality that can be cultivated and improved over time with the right approach and consistent effort. Stretching is one of the most effective ways to enhance flexibility, allowing us to lengthen and loosen tight muscles, improve range of motion in our joints, and reduce the risk of injury during physical activity. In this chapter, we will explore the various types of stretching, safe stretching techniques, and sample stretching routines to help you unlock your body's full potential.

Different Types of Stretching

Stretching comes in many forms, each with its own unique benefits and applications. Understanding the different types of stretching can help you tailor your routine to suit your individual needs and goals. Here are some of the most common types of stretching:

- **Static Stretching**: This is perhaps the most familiar type of stretching, involving holding a stretch position for a prolonged period (usually 15-30 seconds) without movement. Static stretching targets specific muscles or muscle groups and helps improve flexibility by elongating muscle fibers and increasing blood flow to the area. Examples of static stretches include the hamstring stretch, quadriceps stretch, and calf stretch.

- **Dynamic Stretching**: Dynamic stretching involves moving the body through a full range of motion in a controlled manner. Unlike static stretching, which focuses on holding a stretch position, dynamic stretching uses repetitive movements to warm up the muscles and prepare them for physical activity. Dynamic stretches often mimic the movements of the activity you're about to perform and can help improve flexibility, mobility, and athletic performance.

- **Ballistic Stretching**: Ballistic stretching involves using bouncing or jerking movements to force a muscle beyond its normal range of motion. While ballistic stretching can be effective for improving flexibility, it also carries a higher risk of injury, especially if performed incorrectly. For this reason, it's generally not recommended for most individuals, particularly those with limited flexibility or joint issues.

- **Proprioceptive Neuromuscular Facilitation (PNF)**: PNF stretching is a more advanced form of stretching that involves a combination of passive stretching and isometric contractions. PNF techniques often require a partner or a prop, such as a resistance band or wall, to facilitate the stretch. PNF stretching can be highly effective for improving flexibility, as it targets both the muscles and the nervous system, promoting greater gains in range of motion.

- **Yoga and Pilates**: Yoga and Pilates are holistic mind-body practices that incorporate stretching, strength training, and breath work to improve flexibility, balance, and overall well-being. Both disciplines offer a wide range of stretching exercises, from gentle stretches in yoga's hatha tradition to dynamic movements in Pilates' core-focused repertoire. Whether you're a beginner or an experienced practitioner, yoga and Pilates offer something for everyone seeking to enhance flexibility and mobility.

Safe Stretching Techniques

While stretching can be highly beneficial for improving flexibility, it's important to approach it with caution and mindfulness to avoid injury. Here are some safe stretching techniques to keep in mind:

- **Warm-Up First**: Before diving into your stretching routine, it's essential to warm up your muscles with some light aerobic activity, such as walking, jogging, or cycling. Warming up increases blood flow to the muscles, making them more pliable and less susceptible to injury during stretching.

- **Go Slow and Gentle**: When performing static stretches, avoid bouncing or jerking movements, as these can strain the muscles and lead to injury. Instead, ease into each stretch slowly and gently, stopping at the point where you feel a mild tension in the muscle. Hold the stretch for 15-30 seconds, breathing deeply and steadily throughout.

- **Focus on Form**: Pay attention to your body alignment and posture during stretching to ensure proper technique and effectiveness. Keep your movements smooth and controlled, and avoid overarching or straining the muscles beyond their limits. If you feel any sharp or intense pain, ease off the stretch immediately and reassess your approach.

- **Listen to Your Body**: Flexibility varies from person to person, so it's essential to listen to your body and honor its limitations. Avoid comparing yourself to others or pushing yourself too hard, as this can lead to injury and setbacks. Instead, focus on gradual progress and celebrate small victories along the way.

- **Stay Consistent**: Like any form of exercise, consistency is key to seeing results from stretching. Aim to incorporate stretching into your daily routine, whether it's a few minutes in the morning to wake up your body or a longer session after a workout to cool down and relax. By making stretching a regular habit, you'll gradually improve your flexibility and reap the benefits over time.

Sample Stretching Routines

Now that we've covered the basics of stretching and safe stretching techniques, let's put theory into practice with some sample stretching routines. These routines can be customized to suit your individual needs and preferences, whether you're looking to improve flexibility, relieve muscle tension, or enhance recovery after exercise.

- **Full-Body Stretching Routine**:
  1. Start with a brief warm-up, such as 5-10 minutes of light cardio (e.g., jogging in place, jumping jacks).
  2. Perform static stretches for major muscle groups, including the calves, hamstrings, quadriceps, hip flexors, chest, shoulders, and back.
  3. Hold each stretch for 15-30 seconds, breathing deeply and steadily throughout.
  4. Focus on areas of tightness or discomfort, adjusting the intensity of the stretch as needed.

5. Repeat the sequence 2-3 times, gradually increasing the duration and intensity of the stretches as your flexibility improves.

- **Dynamic Stretching Warm-Up**:
    1. Begin with 5-10 minutes of light aerobic activity to warm up the muscles.
    2. Perform dynamic stretches that target major muscle groups, such as leg swings, arm circles, torso twists, and walking lunges.
    3. Move through each stretch smoothly and rhythmically, focusing on controlled movements and full range of motion.
    4. Perform 10-12 repetitions of each dynamic stretch, gradually increasing the intensity as your muscles warm up.
    5. Finish with a few static stretches to target specific areas of tightness or tension, holding each stretch for 15-30 seconds.

- **Post-Workout Stretching Routine**:
    1. Cool down with 5-10 minutes of light aerobic activity to bring your heart rate down and promote circulation.
    2. Focus on static stretches for major muscle groups that were engaged during your workout, such as the quadriceps, hamstrings, glutes, chest, and shoulders.
    3. Hold each stretch for 15-30 seconds, breathing deeply and allowing the muscles to relax and lengthen.

4. Pay special attention to areas of tightness or discomfort, adjusting the intensity of the stretch as needed.

5. Finish with gentle, relaxing stretches for the neck, shoulders, and lower back to release tension and promote relaxation.

BALANCING ACT: THE FUNDAMENTALS

Balance – it's the silent hero of our daily movements, the unsung champion that keeps us steady on our feet and poised for action. In this chapter, we'll explore the fundamental aspects of balance, from why it matters to the intricate systems in the body that govern it, and how you can assess and improve your own balance for a life of stability and vitality.

Why Balance Matters

Balance isn't just about avoiding embarrassing stumbles or executing flawless yoga poses (although those are certainly nice perks); it's a fundamental aspect of movement and functionality that affects virtually every aspect of our lives. Whether you're walking down the street, reaching for a high shelf, or navigating a rocky hiking trail, balance is what keeps us upright, stable, and in control.

But beyond its role in preventing falls and maintaining posture, balance plays a crucial role in athletic performance, injury prevention, and overall well-being. Athletes rely on balance to execute precise movements, change direction quickly, and maintain optimal body control during competition. Additionally, good balance can help reduce the risk of injuries, such as sprains and strains, by enhancing proprioception – the body's awareness of its position in space – and allowing for more efficient movement patterns.

Furthermore, balance is closely linked to core strength and stability, as the muscles of the core play a key role in maintaining balance and proper alignment of the spine and pelvis. By improving balance, you can enhance core strength and stability, leading to better posture, reduced back pain, and improved overall functional capacity.

In everyday life, good balance allows us to perform activities with ease and confidence, whether it's walking up a flight of stairs, carrying groceries, or playing with our children or grandchildren. By prioritizing balance training and incorporating it into our daily routine, we can enjoy a higher quality of life and greater independence as we age.

Balance Systems in the Body

Achieving and maintaining balance is a complex process that involves multiple systems in the body working together seamlessly to keep us steady and stable. Three primary sensory systems contribute to our sense of balance:

1. **Vestibular System**: Located in the inner ear, the vestibular system is responsible for detecting changes in head position and movement. It consists of fluid-filled canals and tiny hair cells that sense motion and relay information to the brain about the body's orientation in space.

2. **Visual System**: Our eyes provide important visual cues that help us maintain balance and spatial orientation. By observing our surroundings and detecting changes in our environment, our visual system helps us adjust our posture and movement to maintain stability.

3. **Somatosensory System**: This system includes receptors in the muscles, joints, and skin that provide feedback to the brain about the position and movement of the body. By sensing pressure,

tension, and other tactile sensations, the somatosensory system helps us maintain balance and coordination during various activities.

These three sensory systems work together in a coordinated fashion to provide the brain with information about our body's position and movement in space. When one system is compromised or impaired – such as in cases of inner ear dysfunction or vision loss – the other systems compensate to maintain balance and stability.

Assessing Your Balance

Assessing your balance is an important first step in identifying areas of weakness or instability and developing a targeted balance training program. While there are many ways to assess balance, here are a few simple tests you can try at home:

1. **Single Leg Balance Test**: Stand on one leg with your hands on your hips and lift your opposite foot off the ground. Hold this position for 30 seconds, keeping your hips level and your standing knee slightly bent. Repeat on the other leg and compare your performance on each side.

2. **Tandem Stance Test**: Stand with one foot directly in front of the other, heel to toe, with your arms crossed over your chest. Hold this position for 30 seconds, maintaining your balance without swaying or touching the ground. Repeat with the opposite foot in front.

3. **Reach Test**: Stand with your feet hip-width apart and reach forward as far as you can without losing your balance or taking a

step. Measure the distance you can reach and compare it to normative values for your age and gender.

4. **Dynamic Balance Test**: Perform dynamic movements that challenge your balance, such as walking heel to toe in a straight line, standing up from a seated position without using your hands, or walking on uneven terrain (e.g., grass, sand).

By regularly assessing your balance and monitoring your progress over time, you can identify areas of improvement and track the effectiveness of your balance training program. Additionally, seeking guidance from a qualified fitness professional or physical therapist can provide valuable insights and personalized recommendations for improving balance and reducing the risk of falls and injuries.

balance is a fundamental aspect of movement and functionality that affects virtually every aspect of our lives. By understanding the importance of balance, the systems in the body that govern it, and how to assess and improve our own balance, we can enhance our stability, confidence, and overall quality of life. Whether you're an athlete looking to improve performance or an older adult seeking to maintain independence and vitality, prioritizing balance training can have profound benefits for your health and well-being.

EXERCISES FOR IMPROVED BALANCE

Incorporating balance exercises into your fitness routine is a surefire way to enhance stability, coordination, and overall physical well-being. Whether you're a novice or a seasoned athlete, balance training offers a myriad of benefits for individuals of all fitness levels. In this chapter, we'll explore the principles of balance training, provide a range of beginner, intermediate, and advanced balance exercises, and offer tips for incorporating balance into your daily routine for lasting results.

Balance Training Principles

Before diving into specific exercises, let's first establish some fundamental principles of balance training. These principles serve as a guiding framework for designing an effective and safe balance training program:

- **Progressive Overload**: Like any form of exercise, balance training requires progressive overload to stimulate adaptation and improvement. Start with basic exercises and gradually increase the difficulty or intensity over time as your balance improves.

- **Variety and Variation**: Incorporate a variety of balance exercises that target different muscle groups and movement patterns. This not only keeps your workouts interesting and engaging but also ensures balanced development and reduces the risk of overuse injuries.

- **Stability and Control**: Focus on maintaining stability and control throughout each exercise, rather than rushing through the movements. Quality of movement is paramount in balance training, so prioritize proper form and technique over quantity or speed.

- **Challenge and Adaptation**: Challenge yourself with exercises that push you out of your comfort zone and force you to adapt and grow. Experiment with different surfaces, props, and variations to continuously challenge your balance and prevent plateaus.

- **Integration and Coordination**: Balance training is not just about standing on one leg; it's about integrating balance into functional movements and activities of daily living. Look for exercises that mimic real-life situations and require coordination between multiple muscle groups and joints.

By following these principles, you can design a balanced and effective balance training program that addresses your individual needs and goals while minimizing the risk of injury and maximizing results.

Beginner, Intermediate, and Advanced Balance Exercises

Now, let's explore a range of balance exercises suitable for individuals of all fitness levels, from beginners to advanced practitioners:

1. **Beginner Exercises**:
    - Single Leg Balance: Stand on one leg while keeping the other foot slightly off the ground. Hold this position for 15-30 seconds, focusing on stability and control. Repeat on the other leg.
    - Tandem Stance: Stand with one foot directly in front of the other, heel to toe, and hold this position for 15-30

seconds. Keep your arms relaxed at your sides and maintain a tall posture.

- Static Balance Board: Stand on a balance board or wobble board with feet hip-width apart and knees slightly bent. Hold onto a stable surface if necessary and try to maintain balance for 30-60 seconds.

2. **Intermediate Exercises**:

- Dynamic Single Leg Balance: Stand on one leg and perform small knee bends or hip circles while maintaining balance. Focus on smooth, controlled movements and avoid touching the ground with the other foot.

- Bosu Ball Squats: Stand on a Bosu ball with feet hip-width apart and perform squats by bending your knees and lowering your hips toward the ground. Keep your core engaged and maintain balance throughout the movement.

- Foam Roller Balancing: Stand on a foam roller with feet hip-width apart and knees slightly bent. Engage your core muscles to stabilize your body as the roller moves beneath you. Start with small movements and gradually increase the challenge.

3. **Advanced Exercises**:

- Single Leg Romanian Deadlifts: Stand on one leg while holding a dumbbell or kettlebell in one hand. Hinge at the hips and lower the weight toward the ground while extending your free leg behind you for balance. Return to the starting position and repeat on the other leg.

- Stability Ball Planks: Place your forearms on a stability ball and extend your legs behind you into a plank position. Engage your core muscles to stabilize your body and hold the position for 30-60 seconds.

- Yoga Tree Pose: Stand on one leg and bring the sole of the opposite foot to rest against the inner thigh or calf of the standing leg. Press your palms together in front of your chest and hold the pose for 30-60 seconds. Repeat on the other side.

Incorporating Balance into Your Daily Routine

Balance training doesn't have to be limited to the gym; you can incorporate balance exercises into your daily routine to improve stability, coordination, and overall physical function. Here are some simple ways to sneak balance training into your day-to-day activities:

- **Standing on One Leg**: Practice standing on one leg while brushing your teeth, waiting in line, or cooking dinner.

- **Balancing on Unstable Surfaces**: Stand on a cushion, folded towel, or foam pad while performing household chores or watching TV.

- **Taking the Stairs**: Use the stairs instead of the elevator whenever possible to challenge your balance and engage your leg muscles.

- **Walking on Uneven Terrain**: Take a nature walk or hike on uneven terrain to improve proprioception and balance.

- **Using Balance Tools**: Incorporate balance tools such as stability balls, balance boards, or foam rollers into your workouts or stretching routines.

By integrating balance exercises into your daily routine, you can gradually improve stability, coordination, and proprioception while simultaneously enhancing your overall fitness and well-being.

In conclusion, balance training is a valuable component of any fitness program, offering a wide range of benefits for individuals of all fitness levels. By following the principles of balance training, incorporating a variety of exercises, and finding creative ways to integrate balance into your daily routine, you can enhance stability, coordination, and overall physical function for a life of vitality and well-being. Whether you're a beginner looking to improve balance or an advanced practitioner seeking new challenges, there's a balance exercise suitable for everyone.

FLEXIBILITY AND BALANCE ACROSS THE LIFESPAN

Flexibility and balance are not static qualities; they evolve and change as we journey through the different stages of life. From the exuberance of childhood to the wisdom of old age, maintaining optimal flexibility and balance is essential for overall well-being and functional independence. In this chapter, we'll explore how flexibility and balance evolve across the lifespan, from childhood to older adulthood, and provide strategies for promoting and preserving these vital components of physical health.

Flexibility and Balance in Children

Children are natural movers, constantly exploring their environment and pushing the boundaries of their physical abilities. Flexibility and balance play a crucial role in children's motor development, allowing them to navigate the world with confidence and grace.

During childhood, flexibility is at its peak, thanks to the natural elasticity of muscles and connective tissues. Children effortlessly perform feats of flexibility, such as bending over to touch their toes or contorting their bodies into playful yoga poses. This innate flexibility not only allows children to explore their physical potential but also supports the development of motor skills and coordination.

Similarly, balance is a foundational skill that children begin to develop from infancy. As they learn to sit up, crawl, and eventually walk, children rely on balance to maintain stability and control their movements. Activities such as climbing, jumping, and riding a bike further challenge and refine their balance skills, laying the groundwork for more complex movements and activities later in life.

Encouraging active play and participation in sports and physical activities is essential for promoting flexibility and balance in children. Activities that involve stretching, reaching, and balancing help improve flexibility and proprioception while enhancing coordination and motor skills. By fostering a supportive environment that encourages movement and exploration, parents and caregivers can help children develop a lifelong love of physical activity and a strong foundation of flexibility and balance.

Flexibility and Balance in Adolescents and Young Adults

As children transition into adolescence and young adulthood, the demands on their bodies evolve, and so too does their relationship with flexibility and balance. During this stage of life, flexibility may begin to decline slightly as the body undergoes rapid growth and maturation. Muscles and connective tissues may become tighter and less pliable, particularly in response to prolonged periods of sitting and sedentary behavior.

However, with regular physical activity and targeted flexibility training, adolescents and young adults can maintain and even improve their flexibility over time. Incorporating activities such as yoga, Pilates, and dynamic stretching into their fitness routine can help counteract the effects of sedentary behavior and promote healthy movement patterns.

Balance also continues to be important during adolescence and young adulthood, particularly as individuals engage in more complex physical activities and sports. Activities that challenge balance, such as surfing, skateboarding, and martial arts, not only improve proprioception and coordination but also enhance cognitive function and decision-making skills.

Encouraging adolescents and young adults to participate in a variety of physical activities and sports can help them develop a well-rounded skill set that includes flexibility, balance, strength, and endurance. By fostering a holistic approach to fitness and movement, young individuals can lay the foundation for a lifetime of health and vitality.

Maintaining Flexibility and Balance in Middle Age

As individuals enter middle age, the importance of flexibility and balance becomes even more apparent, particularly as the body begins to experience the effects of aging. Muscle mass may decrease, joints may become stiffer, and balance may become less steady, increasing the risk of falls and injuries.

However, middle age is not a time to resign oneself to decreased flexibility and balance; rather, it's an opportunity to prioritize these aspects of physical health and well-being. Regular exercise, including activities that promote flexibility and balance, becomes essential for maintaining mobility, preventing injuries, and preserving independence. Incorporating activities such as yoga, Tai Chi, and flexibility training into a fitness routine can help counteract the effects of aging on flexibility and balance. These low-impact activities not only improve flexibility and balance but also promote relaxation, stress reduction, and overall well-being.

Additionally, strength training exercises that target the core, lower body, and stabilizing muscles can enhance balance and stability, reducing the risk of falls and improving functional capacity. By adopting a well-rounded approach to fitness that includes flexibility, balance, strength, and cardiovascular training, individuals can mitigate the effects of aging on their physical health and maintain an active and vibrant lifestyle.

Flexibility and Balance Considerations for Older Adults

As individuals enter older adulthood, flexibility and balance become increasingly important for maintaining independence, preventing falls, and enhancing quality of life. Aging is often accompanied by changes in flexibility and balance, including decreased muscle mass, joint stiffness, and diminished proprioception.

However, with proper care and attention, older adults can continue to improve and maintain flexibility and balance well into their later years. Incorporating gentle stretching exercises, such as yoga, Tai Chi, and Pilates, into a daily routine can help improve flexibility, reduce stiffness, and enhance range of motion in older adults.

Balance training exercises that focus on stability, coordination, and proprioception are also essential for older adults. Activities such as standing on one leg, walking heel-to-toe, and practicing balance exercises on unstable surfaces (e.g., foam pads, balance boards) can help improve balance and reduce the risk of falls.

Moreover, strength training exercises that target the major muscle groups, particularly those involved in posture and balance, can help improve overall stability and functional capacity in older adults. Exercises such as squats, lunges, and calf raises can help strengthen the lower body and improve balance and mobility.

It's also important for older adults to address any underlying medical conditions or physical limitations that may affect flexibility and balance. Working with a qualified healthcare professional or physical therapist can provide guidance and personalized recommendations for improving flexibility and balance while minimizing the risk of injury.

In conclusion, flexibility and balance are essential components of physical health and well-being that evolve across the lifespan. From childhood to older adulthood, maintaining optimal flexibility and balance is key to promoting independence, preventing falls, and enhancing overall quality of life. By incorporating regular physical activity, targeted flexibility and balance exercises, and personalized interventions as needed, individuals can enjoy a lifetime of health, vitality, and mobility.

SPECIAL CONSIDERATIONS AND ADAPTATIONS

Flexibility and balance are essential components of physical health and well-being that can benefit individuals from all walks of life. However, certain populations may face unique challenges or considerations when it comes to maintaining and improving flexibility and balance. In this chapter, we'll explore special considerations and adaptations for individuals with disabilities, during pregnancy, and for athletes, providing strategies and recommendations tailored to each group's specific needs.

Flexibility and Balance for Individuals with Disabilities

For individuals with disabilities, flexibility and balance can play a crucial role in enhancing mobility, independence, and overall quality of life. However, navigating the realm of flexibility and balance training may require adaptations and modifications to accommodate different abilities and challenges.

One key consideration for individuals with disabilities is to focus on exercises and activities that are safe, accessible, and appropriate for their specific needs and abilities. This may involve working with a qualified healthcare professional, physical therapist, or adaptive fitness trainer who can provide guidance and personalized recommendations.

For individuals with mobility impairments or wheelchair users, seated stretching exercises can help improve flexibility in the upper body, shoulders, and spine. Utilizing resistance bands or yoga straps can assist with stretching while seated and provide support for individuals with limited mobility.

Similarly, balance training exercises can be adapted to accommodate individuals with disabilities, such as using stable surfaces or support bars for stability and safety. Seated balance exercises, such as seated leg lifts or seated side bends, can help improve core strength and stability while minimizing the risk of falls.

In addition to physical adaptations, it's essential to consider the psychological and emotional aspects of flexibility and balance training for individuals with disabilities. Providing a supportive and inclusive environment that fosters confidence, autonomy, and self-efficacy can empower individuals to embrace their unique abilities and achieve their fitness goals.

Flexibility and Balance during Pregnancy

Pregnancy is a time of profound physical and hormonal changes that can impact flexibility and balance. As the body prepares for childbirth, ligaments become more relaxed, joints may become looser, and the center of gravity shifts, affecting balance and stability.

During pregnancy, it's essential to prioritize safe and gentle forms of flexibility and balance training that accommodate the body's changing needs and limitations. Avoiding high-impact activities and exercises that put excessive strain on the joints and ligaments is crucial to minimize the risk of injury.

Prenatal yoga and Pilates are excellent options for maintaining flexibility and improving balance during pregnancy. These low-impact exercises focus on gentle stretching, controlled movements, and breath work, providing a safe and effective way to stay active and mobile while supporting the changing needs of the body.

Incorporating pelvic floor exercises, such as Kegels, into a prenatal fitness routine can also help improve pelvic stability and support during pregnancy and childbirth. These exercises strengthen the muscles of the pelvic floor, which play a vital role in maintaining bladder control, supporting the uterus, and facilitating childbirth.

As pregnancy progresses, it's essential to listen to your body and adjust your exercise routine accordingly. Avoiding exercises that involve lying flat on your back or putting pressure on the abdomen after the first trimester is important to prevent complications such as decreased blood flow to the uterus.

Consulting with a prenatal fitness specialist or healthcare provider can provide personalized guidance and recommendations for maintaining flexibility and balance during pregnancy. By staying active, practicing safe stretching and balance exercises, and listening to your body's cues, you can support your physical and emotional well-being throughout pregnancy and beyond.

Flexibility and Balance for Athletes

Athletes, whether professional or recreational, rely on flexibility and balance to optimize performance, prevent injuries, and maintain peak physical condition. Incorporating targeted flexibility and balance training into an athlete's regimen can enhance agility, coordination, and overall athletic performance.

For athletes, flexibility is essential for achieving optimal range of motion in joints and muscles, allowing for fluid and efficient movement patterns.

Dynamic stretching exercises that mimic the movements of the sport or activity can help prepare the body for action while improving flexibility and mobility.

Balance training is equally important for athletes, as it enhances proprioception, spatial awareness, and neuromuscular control – all of which are essential for agility, coordination, and injury prevention. Incorporating balance exercises such as single-leg squats, stability ball exercises, and agility drills into a training program can help improve balance and stability on and off the field.

In addition to traditional flexibility and balance training, athletes may benefit from incorporating other modalities such as foam rolling, massage therapy, and mobility drills into their routine. These techniques can help alleviate muscle tension, improve tissue quality, and enhance overall flexibility and range of motion.

It's important for athletes to pay attention to their body's feedback and adjust their training program accordingly to prevent overuse injuries and promote recovery. Incorporating rest days, cross-training activities, and active recovery strategies can help maintain a balance between training intensity and recovery, allowing for continued progress and performance gains.

Furthermore, athletes should prioritize proper nutrition, hydration, and sleep to support optimal recovery and performance. Adequate intake of protein, carbohydrates, healthy fats, vitamins, and minerals is essential for supporting muscle repair, replenishing energy stores, and promoting overall health and well-being.

In conclusion, flexibility and balance are integral components of physical health and performance for individuals with disabilities, during pregnancy, and for athletes. By understanding the unique needs and considerations of each population and adapting training strategies accordingly, individuals can optimize flexibility, improve balance, and enhance overall well-being and quality of life. Whether it's making modifications for accessibility, adjusting routines for pregnancy, or fine-tuning training programs for athletic performance, flexibility and balance training can be tailored to meet the diverse needs and goals of individuals across all walks of life.

LIFESTYLE FACTORS FOR OPTIMAL FLEXIBILITY AND BALANCE

Achieving and maintaining optimal flexibility and balance isn't just about the exercises you do in the gym; it's also influenced by various lifestyle factors that impact your overall health and well-being. In this chapter, we'll delve into the importance of nutrition and hydration, sleep and recovery, and stress management for promoting optimal flexibility and balance, providing practical strategies and recommendations for integrating these lifestyle factors into your daily routine.

Nutrition and Hydration

Nutrition and hydration are cornerstones of overall health and well-being, playing a vital role in supporting physical performance, recovery, and muscle function. When it comes to flexibility and balance, proper nutrition and hydration are equally important, providing the essential nutrients and fluids needed to support muscle flexibility, joint health, and overall physical function.

A balanced diet rich in nutrient-dense foods such as fruits, vegetables, whole grains, lean proteins, and healthy fats is essential for supporting flexibility and balance. These foods provide the vitamins, minerals, antioxidants, and phytonutrients that support muscle health, reduce inflammation, and promote tissue repair and regeneration.

In particular, certain nutrients play a key role in maintaining flexibility and joint health. For example, vitamin D is essential for calcium absorption and bone health, while omega-3 fatty acids found in fish oil have anti-inflammatory properties that can help reduce joint pain and stiffness.

Additionally, staying well-hydrated is crucial for maintaining optimal flexibility and balance. Dehydration can lead to muscle cramps, fatigue, and reduced joint lubrication, making it more challenging to perform exercises and activities that require flexibility and coordination. Aim to drink plenty of water throughout the day, especially before, during, and after exercise, to stay hydrated and support muscle function and recovery.

Incorporating foods rich in electrolytes such as potassium, magnesium, and sodium can also help maintain fluid balance and support muscle function. Examples include bananas, leafy greens, nuts, seeds, and electrolyte-rich sports drinks.

Finally, paying attention to meal timing and composition can also impact flexibility and balance. Consuming a balanced meal or snack containing carbohydrates and protein before and after exercise can provide the necessary energy and nutrients to support muscle function and recovery. Aim to eat a variety of nutrient-dense foods throughout the day to support overall health and well-being while also promoting optimal flexibility and balance.

Sleep and Recovery

Quality sleep and adequate recovery are essential components of any successful fitness program, including those focused on improving flexibility and balance. During sleep, the body undergoes essential processes such as tissue repair, muscle growth, and hormone regulation, all of which are crucial for supporting physical performance and recovery.

For optimal flexibility and balance, aim to prioritize sleep and establish a consistent sleep routine that allows for adequate rest and recovery. Most adults require 7-9 hours of sleep per night to function optimally, although individual needs may vary.

Creating a sleep-friendly environment can help improve sleep quality and promote relaxation before bedtime. Make sure your bedroom is dark, quiet, and cool, and avoid screens and stimulating activities before bedtime. Establishing a relaxing bedtime routine, such as reading, listening to calming music, or practicing relaxation techniques, can also help prepare the body and mind for sleep.

In addition to sleep, incorporating rest and recovery days into your workout routine is essential for preventing overtraining and promoting muscle repair and regeneration. Listen to your body's cues and give yourself permission to rest and recover when needed, whether it's taking a day off from intense exercise or incorporating active recovery activities such as walking, yoga, or stretching into your routine.

Massage therapy, foam rolling, and other recovery techniques can also help alleviate muscle tension, reduce soreness, and improve flexibility and range of motion. These techniques promote blood flow to the muscles, which can aid in the removal of metabolic waste products and support tissue repair and recovery.

Finally, paying attention to stress management and mental well-being is essential for promoting quality sleep and optimal recovery. Chronic stress can disrupt sleep patterns, increase muscle tension, and impair recovery, negatively impacting flexibility and balance. Incorporating stress-reducing activities such as meditation, deep breathing exercises, or mindfulness practices into your daily routine can help promote relaxation, improve sleep quality, and support overall physical and mental health.

Stress Management

Stress is a common and often unavoidable part of modern life, but managing stress effectively is essential for promoting optimal flexibility and balance. Chronic stress can have a profound impact on the body, leading to muscle tension, impaired recovery, and reduced flexibility and balance.

One of the most effective ways to manage stress is through regular physical activity and exercise. Exercise has been shown to reduce levels of stress hormones such as cortisol while increasing the production of endorphins, neurotransmitters that promote feelings of well-being and relaxation. Engaging in activities such as yoga, Pilates, or tai chi can be particularly effective for reducing stress and promoting relaxation while also improving flexibility and balance.

In addition to physical activity, incorporating stress-reducing techniques such as meditation, deep breathing exercises, and progressive muscle relaxation into your daily routine can help promote relaxation and reduce muscle tension. These techniques help activate the body's relaxation response, counteracting the physiological effects of stress and promoting a sense of calm and tranquility.

Furthermore, fostering social connections and maintaining a strong support network can help buffer the effects of stress and promote emotional well-being. Spending time with friends and loved ones, engaging in meaningful activities, and seeking support from others can provide a sense of belonging and connection that helps reduce stress and improve overall resilience.

Finally, practicing self-care and prioritizing activities that bring joy and fulfillment can help reduce stress and promote overall well-being. Whether it's spending time in nature, pursuing hobbies and interests, or simply taking time for yourself, making self-care a priority can help recharge your batteries and improve your ability to cope with stress.

In conclusion, lifestyle factors such as nutrition and hydration, sleep and recovery, and stress management play a critical role in promoting optimal flexibility and balance. By prioritizing these aspects of health and well-being and incorporating practical strategies into your daily routine, you can support your body's natural ability to move, perform, and thrive. Whether it's fueling your body with nutrient-dense foods, prioritizing quality sleep and recovery, or practicing stress-reducing techniques, taking care of your body and mind is essential for achieving and maintaining optimal flexibility and balance throughout life.

INJURY PREVENTION AND REHABILITATION

Injuries can be a significant setback when it comes to maintaining flexibility and balance. Whether you're an athlete pushing your limits or someone looking to improve your overall physical well-being, injuries can hinder progress and disrupt your routine. However, with the right knowledge and approach, you can take steps to prevent injuries and effectively rehabilitate if they occur.

Common Flexibility and Balance-Related Injuries

Flexibility and balance training are generally low-impact activities, but injuries can still occur, especially when proper form and technique are not observed, or when pushing beyond one's limits. Some of the most common injuries related to flexibility and balance training include:

- **Muscle Strains and Sprains**: Overstretching or sudden movements can result in muscle strains or sprains, which involve the stretching or tearing of muscle fibers or ligaments.

- **Joint Injuries**: Twisting or hyperextending joints beyond their normal range of motion can lead to injuries such as dislocations, subluxations, or ligament tears.

- **Overuse Injuries**: Repetitive movements or excessive training without adequate rest can result in overuse injuries, such as tendinitis or stress fractures.

- **Falls**: Loss of balance during exercises or activities can lead to falls, resulting in injuries such as bruises, fractures, or head injuries.

Understanding the common types of injuries related to flexibility and balance training can help you take proactive steps to prevent them and minimize their impact on your overall well-being.

Strategies for Preventing Injuries

Prevention is key when it comes to avoiding injuries related to flexibility and balance training. By implementing the following strategies, you can reduce the risk of injury and maintain a safe and effective workout routine:

- **Warm-Up Properly**: Always start your workout with a thorough warm-up to prepare your muscles, joints, and connective tissues for activity. Incorporate dynamic stretches and movements that mimic the exercises you'll be performing during your workout.

- **Gradually Increase Intensity**: Avoid overexertion by gradually increasing the intensity, duration, and complexity of your flexibility and balance exercises over time. Listen to your body's cues and avoid pushing through pain or discomfort.

- **Focus on Proper Form**: Pay close attention to your form and technique during exercises to ensure proper alignment and reduce the risk of injury. Engage your core muscles, maintain neutral spine alignment, and avoid jerky or sudden movements.

- **Use Appropriate Equipment**: Choose equipment and gear that are suitable for your skill level and activity. Invest in supportive footwear, appropriate clothing, and any necessary safety equipment to reduce the risk of injury during exercise.

- **Incorporate Variety**: Avoid overuse injuries by incorporating a variety of exercises and activities into your flexibility and balance training routine. Cross-training with different modalities can help prevent repetitive strain on specific muscles and joints.

- **Listen to Your Body**: Pay attention to warning signs such as pain, discomfort, or fatigue, and adjust your workout accordingly. Rest and recover when needed, and don't hesitate to seek medical attention if you experience persistent or severe pain.

By implementing these strategies into your flexibility and balance training routine, you can reduce the risk of injury and maintain a safe and effective workout regimen.

Rehabilitation Approaches

Despite your best efforts, injuries may still occur from time to time. When injuries do happen, it's essential to take a proactive approach to rehabilitation to promote healing, restore function, and prevent re-injury. Here are some key approaches to rehabilitation for common flexibility and balance-related injuries:

- **Rest and Recovery**: In the immediate aftermath of an injury, it's crucial to allow time for rest and recovery to prevent further damage and promote healing. Avoid activities that exacerbate pain or discomfort and focus on gentle movements and stretches that promote circulation and mobility.

- **R.I.C.E. Protocol**: The R.I.C.E. protocol (Rest, Ice, Compression, Elevation) is a common approach to managing acute injuries such as strains, sprains, or bruises. Rest the injured area, apply ice to reduce swelling, use compression bandages to support the injured area, and elevate the injured limb above heart level to reduce swelling and promote circulation.

- **Physical Therapy**: Working with a physical therapist can be instrumental in guiding your rehabilitation journey, providing personalized exercises, stretches, and techniques to promote healing and restore function. Physical therapy may include a combination of manual therapy, therapeutic exercises, and modalities such as heat, ice, or electrical stimulation.

- **Gradual Return to Activity**: As the injured area begins to heal, gradually reintroduce activity and exercise under the guidance of a healthcare professional. Start with gentle movements and low-impact exercises, gradually increasing intensity and duration as tolerated.

- **Strength and Stability Training**: Incorporate strength and stability exercises into your rehabilitation program to rebuild muscle strength, improve joint stability, and prevent future injuries. Focus on targeting the muscles surrounding the injured area while maintaining proper form and alignment.

- **Flexibility and Mobility Work**: Include flexibility and mobility exercises to restore range of motion and flexibility in the injured area. Gentle stretching, foam rolling, and mobility drills can help reduce stiffness and improve function.

- **Mind-Body Techniques**: Incorporate mind-body techniques such as yoga, meditation, or deep breathing exercises to reduce stress, promote relaxation, and enhance overall well-being during the rehabilitation process.

By taking a comprehensive approach to rehabilitation that addresses both the physical and psychological aspects of injury recovery, you can expedite healing, restore function, and minimize the risk of re-injury. It's essential to be patient and consistent with your rehabilitation efforts, allowing your body the time and support it needs to fully recover and return to your desired level of activity. If you have any questions or concerns about your injury or rehabilitation program, don't hesitate to consult with a qualified healthcare professional for guidance and support.

CREATING YOUR FLEXIBILITY AND BALANCE PLAN

Achieving optimal flexibility and balance requires more than just performing a few stretches or balance exercises here and there. To truly make progress and see results, you need a well-thought-out plan that addresses your goals, incorporates effective workout routines, and tracks your progress along the way. In this chapter, we'll explore how to put together a comprehensive flexibility and balance plan by setting goals, designing your workout routine, and tracking your progress.

Setting Goals

Setting clear and achievable goals is the first step in creating a successful flexibility and balance plan. Your goals will serve as the roadmap for your journey, guiding your efforts and keeping you motivated along the way. When setting goals for flexibility and balance, consider the following factors:

- **Specificity**: Clearly define what you want to achieve with your flexibility and balance training. Whether it's touching your toes without discomfort, mastering a challenging yoga pose, or improving your balance to prevent falls, make sure your goals are specific and measurable.

- **Realistic Expectations**: Set realistic and achievable goals based on your current fitness level, lifestyle, and commitments. While it's important to challenge yourself, setting overly ambitious goals can lead to frustration and burnout. Start with small, attainable goals and gradually increase the difficulty as you progress.

- **Relevance**: Make sure your goals are relevant to your overall health and well-being. Consider how improving flexibility and balance will enhance your quality of life and support your other fitness goals. Whether it's improving athletic performance, reducing pain and stiffness, or enhancing mobility, your goals should align with your values and priorities.

- **Timeline**: Establish a timeline for achieving your goals, breaking them down into short-term and long-term objectives. This will help keep you accountable and provide a sense of direction as you work towards your desired outcomes. Be flexible with your timeline and adjust as needed based on your progress and circumstances.

Once you've established your goals, write them down and revisit them regularly to stay focused and motivated. Celebrate your progress along the way, and don't be afraid to adjust your goals as you learn and grow throughout your flexibility and balance journey.

Designing Your Workout Routine

With your goals in mind, it's time to design a workout routine that will help you achieve them. A well-rounded flexibility and balance routine should include a variety of exercises and activities that target different muscle groups and movement patterns. Here are some key components to consider when designing your workout routine:

- **Flexibility Exercises**: Incorporate a variety of stretching exercises that target major muscle groups and improve overall flexibility. Include static stretches, dynamic stretches, and proprioceptive neuromuscular facilitation (PNF) techniques to enhance range of motion and reduce muscle tension.

- **Balance Exercises**: Include balance exercises that challenge stability, proprioception, and coordination. Exercises such as single-leg stance, balance board drills, and yoga poses can help improve balance and reduce the risk of falls.

- **Strength Training**: Incorporate strength training exercises that complement your flexibility and balance goals. Focus on functional movements that engage multiple muscle groups and improve overall stability and strength. Include exercises such as squats, lunges, push-ups, and plans to build muscle and support joint health.

- **Cardiovascular Exercise**: Don't forget to include cardiovascular exercise in your routine to improve cardiovascular health and endurance. Activities such as walking, jogging, cycling, or swimming can help improve circulation, enhance energy levels, and support overall well-being.

- **Rest and Recovery**: Remember to incorporate rest days into your workout routine to allow your body time to recover and adapt to the demands of exercise. Listen to your body's cues and avoid overtraining, which can increase the risk of injury and hinder progress.

When designing your workout routine, consider your schedule, preferences, and fitness level. Aim for a balanced mix of flexibility, balance, strength, and cardiovascular exercise, and don't be afraid to experiment with different exercises and formats to keep your routine fun and engaging.

Tracking Progress

Tracking your progress is essential for staying motivated and measuring the effectiveness of your flexibility and balance plan. By monitoring your progress regularly, you can identify areas of improvement, track your achievements, and make adjustments as needed to stay on track towards your goals. Here are some effective ways to track your progress:

- **Keep a Workout Journal**: Record your workouts, including the exercises performed, sets, reps, and any notes or observations about your performance. Keeping a workout journal allows you to track your progress over time and identify patterns or trends in your training.

- **Measure Flexibility and Range of Motion**: Use objective measures such as goniometry or flexibility tests to assess your flexibility and range of motion at regular intervals. Keep track of your measurements over time to monitor improvements and identify areas for further focus.

- **Assess Balance and Stability**: Incorporate balance assessments such as single-leg stance tests or stability challenges to evaluate your balance and stability. Record your performance and track changes over time to gauge progress and adjust your training accordingly.

- **Set Milestones and Benchmarks**: Break down your goals into smaller milestones or benchmarks that you can work towards on a regular basis. Celebrate each milestone as you achieve it, and use them as motivation to keep pushing forward towards your ultimate goals.

- **Listen to Your Body**: Pay attention to how your body feels during and after exercise, and adjust your training accordingly. If you experience pain, discomfort, or fatigue, take a step back and reassess your approach to training. Remember that progress is not always linear, and it's okay to take breaks or modify your routine as needed.

Remember to celebrate your achievements along the way, and don't be afraid to seek support and guidance from fitness professionals or healthcare providers if you need assistance with your training program. With dedication, perseverance, and a well-designed plan, you can improve your flexibility and balance and enhance your overall health and well-being for years to come.

CONCLUSION

In conclusion, the journey to optimal flexibility and balance is multifaceted, encompassing various aspects of physical fitness, lifestyle choices, and personal commitment. Throughout this guide, we've explored the importance of flexibility and balance for overall health and well-being, delving into the science behind these concepts, practical strategies for improvement, and considerations for different populations and scenarios.

Flexibility and balance are not just physical attributes; they are also reflections of our overall health and vitality. By prioritizing flexibility and balance in our daily lives, we can enhance our mobility, reduce the risk of injury, and improve our quality of life at any age.

We've learned that flexibility and balance are dynamic qualities that can be improved with consistent practice and attention. Whether you're a seasoned athlete, a busy parent, or someone looking to enhance your overall fitness, there are strategies and approaches that can help you achieve your goals and live life to the fullest.

From setting clear and achievable goals to designing a well-rounded workout routine and tracking your progress along the way, we've explored practical steps you can take to incorporate flexibility and balance training into your life. By taking a holistic approach that considers factors such as nutrition, sleep, stress management, and injury prevention, you can optimize your flexibility and balance and support your overall health and well-being.

As you embark on your flexibility and balance journey, remember that progress takes time and patience. Be kind to yourself and celebrate your achievements along the way, no matter how small they may seem. Stay consistent with your efforts, listen to your body, and be open to adapting your approach as needed.

In the words of Mahatma Gandhi, "It is health that is real wealth and not pieces of gold and silver." Your health is your most precious asset, and investing in your flexibility and balance is an investment in your overall well-being. So, take the first step today towards a healthier, more balanced life, and let the journey unfold with each stretch, each breath, and each mindful step forward. Your body, mind, and spirit will thank you for it.

Remember, your journey towards better health and vitality begins with a single step. Take that step today and watch as your flexibility and balance improve, your energy levels soar, and your zest for life reignites. You have the power to transform your health and create a life filled with vitality, strength, and joy.